MEMORY IMPROVEMENT FOR KIDS

THE GREATEST COLLECTION OF PROVEN TECHNIQUES FOR EXPANDING YOUR CHILD'S MIND AND BOOSTING THEIR BRAIN POWER

LISA MARSHALL

Lisa Marshall

CONTENTS

FREE GIFT

Thank you for purchasing this book! Click on the link to download your FREE gift!

https://bit.ly/childlearningstylez

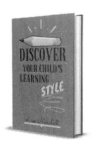

By understanding your child's preferred learning style you can:

- Improve your child's accomplishments and feelings of achievement

- Teach your child coping skills for situations that are not geared to their learning style
- Help your child at home thanks to the best tools

And much more!

DO YOU ENJOY AUDIOBOOKS ?

If you prefer to learn by listening, be sure to check out my audiobooks! You can listen for FREE if you're a first time Audible user as part of their free 30-day trial.

Click the link and enjoy your next audiobook!

https://bit.ly/enjoyaudiobooks

"Unless we remember, we cannot understand"

E.M. FORSTER

INTRODUCTION

Are you looking for ways to improve your child's memory?
Is your child suffering from memory deficit?
Do you desire to raise smart children?

If so, then this book is the solution you need.

With the advent of technology also comes the age of distraction, and with all those technological advances, children are finding it hard to maintain focus and retain thoughts. Traditional methods of teaching lack efficiency to optimize children's learning capability, which results in information overload and memory deficit.

However, there are many ways to help your children get the best of their learning experience and you are the right person to help them enhance their memory. But the question is, how can you achieve that feat?

Research has shown that the brain has the capacity to change and never stops improving through learning (Michelon, 2018). If you feel that your child is not smart enough to quickly grasp the lesson you are trying to teach them, then the issue is not with them, but with YOU!

If you want to raise better children, give them a chance to develop better working memory and help them cultivate their learning prowess.

Research also found that most parents find it hard to relate to their children. This book is designed to help parents get a better understanding of their children by bridging all the gap they find when it comes to relating with them. Often, when it comes to learning, they expect their children to understand them when it should be the other way around.

Memory Improvement for Kids: The Greatest Collection Of Proven Techniques For Expanding Your Child's Mind And Boosting Their Brain Power is geared towards helping parents understand their children better, so they can properly help in providing them with the best learning experience and assist them in getting a better foundation for learning at home.

Your children's education is of vital importance and that's why you invest in their schooling, but I believe that learning institutions and centers are just an extension of your child's learning activities, and their teachers are only facilitating new learning experiences.

The significant part of your child's learning, including brain and behavior foundation, occurs at the very place they spent most of their time: AT HOME.

As a parent, whether you are there or not with them most of the time, you have the responsibility to initiate their learning and memory improvement activities. This should be mandatory if you want to develop smarter and happier children.

Reading this book will provide you with more benefits and they include:

• Exploring your child's world of learning and brain development.

• Determining your child's learning styles and strengths so as to obtain the best results.

• Discovering the basics on how to develop your child's interest in learning.

• Providing your child with the right tools to enhance their IQ.

• Learning how to enhance your child's working memory and retention.

• Ensuring an enjoyable learning environment and maximize their focus.

• Helping your child to develop a growth mindset.

If you think to it better, you will discover that as a parent, you are also learning with your child, but in a different dimension.

After reading this book, I assure you an increase in terms of performances, achievement of better results and a deeper level in your parent-child relationship.

Now, if you are ready to start this journey with your child in the name of brain-boosting, make yourself comfortable and get on reading!

CHAPTER 1

MEMORY AND THE BRAIN

When it comes to the learning process, the brain plays a significant role. Everything starts from the brain, so we must begin our exploration of the human mind.

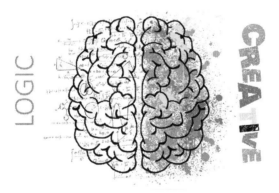

THE ANATOMY OF THE BRAIN

The brain only weighs about three pounds, but it contains our intelligence, controls our senses, and sets our body in motion while directing our behavior.

The human brain consists of three major divisions:

- Forebrain
- Midbrain
- Hindbrain

The **forebrain** is the most significant and highly developed structure in our brain. It is located on the topmost portion of your brain and is associated with all intellectual activities, including memorization, planning, thinking, and visualization.

Activities, like playing with your friends, recognizing someone you have met before, and playing a game are processed in the forebrain.

The **midbrain** is responsible for eye control, reflex actions, and other voluntary movements. It is situated on the topmost part of the brainstem. When you go to a movie, you can experience seeing darkness at first, but as your eyes get adjusted to it, and your pupils dilate to absorb as much light as available, you start to see better. It is because your midbrain is working on this.

Just above your spinal cord is the location of the **hindbrain** that contains the **cerebellum**. This looks like a wrinkled ball of tissue and is responsible for coordinating all your body vital functions and automatic movements. For instance, when doing things that you get used to doing every day like brushing your teeth, writing, or washing your hands, it is the hindbrain that is at work here. It is also the hindbrain that directs the heart rate and respiratory system.

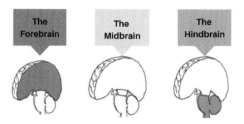

Now let us focus on the cerebellum that sits behind the back of your head. The cerebellum is what provides the balance you need on a bike, skateboard, or surfboard. It is also at play when you touch your nose so you don't poke yourself in the eye.

The cerebellum is also considered the little brain because it looks like a miniature brain on the one just above it.

Here's a little activity for your child to know how their cerebellum works.

Tell your child to stretch out their hands forward or sideward as far as possible. Then ask them to bend their arms, one at a time, and touch their nose using their pointed finger starting with their right hand and then with their left. If they hit their target - which is the NOSE - then they have to thank the cerebellum for doing a good job!

It's the main job of the cerebellum to coordinate your movements, which means that your cerebellum is telling your muscles how to work together in harmony so that your actions are smooth and finely coordinated. The cerebellum is essential in the development of your child's motor activities.

MEMORY AND TYPES OF MEMORY

Memory is the power of the brain to recall stored past experiences or information and retrieve it at a later time.

There are three processes involved in the memory function of the brain according to psychology: encoding, storage, and retrieval.

THE THREE MEMORY PROCESSES

Encoding is the process of receiving, processing, and incorporating the information. Input from outside sources reaches our senses in forms of stimuli - chemical and physical. At this initial stage, information is altered to set the memory for the encoding function.

Storage is the process of creating a permanent record of encoded information. This is the second memory stage where information is maintained and kept.

Retrieval is what we normally call the recognition or the recalling process. We recall back stored information in response to some cue that is needed for certain activities or processes. In this third or final process of memory, we are trying to retrieve information previously stored. Needed information must be located and returned to our consciousness. There are retrieval attempts that may prove to be effortless due to the type of information.

Problems may occur in any of these processes which can lead to memory issues from forgetfulness to amnesia. Distraction can prevent proper encoding of information. At the start, information may not be properly stored or it cannot move from short to long-term storage; and as for the worst, pieces of information stored may not be retrieved at all.

When our brain receives input from outside sources, it stores this information in our memory and there are three major types of memory in our brain where they can be kept. What information, and how long we retain certain information, determine the type of memory in use.

- Sensory Memory
- Short-term Memory
- Long-Term Memory

Sensory Memory

The sensory memory is what remains of our impression of any object as perceived by our senses. Sensory memory allows us to retain impressions of sensory information long after the trigger has ceased. An example of the sensory memory is seeing the fast-moving light in the darkness.

Short-Term Memory

Short-Term Memory enables the brain to remember a minimal amount of information only for a short period.

This part of memory holds only a few items and only lasts for about 20 seconds. Research shows a range of 7 items, + or minus 2, depending on the subject. Short-term memory can be moved to long-term memory through processes like rehearsals. An example is when someone verbally dictates to you a phone number and you're saying it repeatedly to yourself to remember. When someone chooses to intrude on you while you're rehearsing, you may easily forget the information since it is only held by the short-term memory.

Short-term memory is fleeting and can only last for about a second. The best example of this is remembering significant information like a date and a phone number you're trying to take note of while being dictated to. An individual capacity to retain working memory is one of the major predictors of general intelligence that is measured through standard psychological tests.

Under the short-term memory, we have the Working Memory and the Immediate Memory or Rote Memory.

Working Memory

Working memory keeps information in a child's mind for less than a minute. It is a great challenge for our children to move information from their working memories into their long-term memories. If the transfer is not completed within a minute, the information can be lost. So to keep working memory from quickly vanishing into thin air, the information must be able to enter the network of the brain's neuronal structure.

To increase your child's mental manipulation of facts, there are study activities like vocabulary word meanings, and match formulas you may use in your child's learning to retain information as long-term memory without repetition and tedious exercises.

Immediate Memory or Rote Memory

Rote Memory is what is required when learning in school as it involves memorizing facts that are easily forgotten because they are less interesting to the learner, such as a list of vocabulary words. When this list of words isn't paired with interesting connections to make them more meaningful, they are easily forgotten by children. With the absence of neural networks or patterns to connect them, permanent memories are not built.

However, there are learning strategies that can help your child spend less time memorizing including personalizing, motivating, and connecting. What they need to memorize will be much easier when you use activities and strategies to help your children build their learning strengths to efficiently create permanent memories more interestingly and quickly.

Long-Term Memory

Long-term memory is more complex compared to short-term and is further sub-categorized into explicit memory, implicit, and autobiographical.

Explicit Memory or Declarative Memory - This memory requires conscious thought and it is what most of us have in mind when thinking of a memory.

Implicit Memory - In contrast to explicit memory, implicit memory does not require conscious thought as it allows you to do things almost in automation like routine actions.

Autobiographical Memory - We have parts in our life that we can remember more vividly than others, so they usually constitute our biography.

HOW A CHILD'S BRAIN WORKS

When a child is born, his brain is developing more from birth to age 5 than at any other time in a human's life. This early development stage has more impact on the child's learning ability and success in school and later in life. The quality of their experience during the first few years - whether positive or negative, helps shape the development of their brain.

Our brain is known as the command center of the body. A newborn child may have all the neurons that they'll be using their whole life but it is the connection between these neurons that is what makes the brain work. Brain connections enable us to do just about everything, such as thinking, movement, and communication. At least a million synapses or neural connections are made every second.

The brain develops at different rates and its areas are responsible for different abilities. Brain development builds itself up as connections link to each other in different ways and thus helps the child to move and speak as well as rationalize in more complex ways.

To become healthy, responsible, and capable adults, a child's brain must develop these neural connections during their early years. These connections are necessary for higher-level activities such as self-regulation, communication skills, problem solving, and motivation. These skills should be learned at an early age since it is harder for the brain to form such connections later in life.

BUILDING BRAIN CONNECTIONS

Children develop brain connections through their everyday experiences starting from birth. Using their senses to interact with the world, their brain connections are built through positive interactions with their parents and caregivers. A child's daily experience determines which brain connections develop and last for a lifetime from those that don't. This depends on the stimulation and reaction as well as the amount and quality of care that they receive during these early years.

RESPONSIVE AND CARING RELATIONSHIPS

What influences a child's brain development most are the relationships with the adults in their life. A child's healthy brain development must have loving relationships with dependable and responsive adults. These relationships start at home with parents and siblings, then with school and community.

From birth, children serve up invitations for adult interactions either by smiling, cooing or crying. They eventually become more direct during their toddler years by using speaking as a form of communication. This process is fundamental to the child's brain development, so parents, as well as the other people that interact with the child healthily, are contributing to this cause. This is also the reason why children need to play, sing, talk, and read with adults in a nurturing and stable environment.

At birth, a child's brain is just about a quarter of the size of an adult's brain and grows double during the first year. By the age of three, it keeps growing until the size is about 80% the adult size and it is almost 90% the size of an adult's brain in their fifth year.

BUILDING KNOWLEDGE

Until recently, it was believed that a child is born with many brain cells that are irreplaceable and that children came into this world with a set level of intelligence that never changed. But now, it's a clear fact that the brain is a continual work in progress. It is because of the brain's plasticity, or neuroplasticity, that your brain is constantly changing.

This discovery served as the most important neuroscience breakthrough in 400 years. Now, let's understand why brain plasticity is so important and share ways to enhance your brain's plasticity.

NEUROPLASTICITY

Neuroplasticity is derived from the word neuron, which means a nerve cell and plastic which means moldable.

According to a leading pioneer in the science of neuroplasticity, Dr. Michael Mendoza, brain plasticity is the brain's ability to change its neurochemical, anatomical, and functional performance status across the lifespan.

In simple terms, it means that the brain can change. It can form new brain cells and neural connections while improving its capabilities all throughout your life.

The brain continually changes it's structure, chemistry, and functions in response to your thinking and actions. Because our thinking, surroundings, and experiences in life differ, brain plasticity is responsible for making each person's brain unique, This innate capacity to alter has it's profound impact on the development of the brain while you're young and is quite significant in brain growth.

BRAIN PLASTICITY AND EARLY BRAIN DEVELOPMENT

While young, the human brain is malleable. When we are born into this world, we have brains that are large but not formed. But with its large cerebral cortex, the brain is designed to build new neural pathways by learning through experiences.

The brain is rapidly developing during the first few years but as we approach the adolescent stage, a lot of information that is considered unimportant is weeded out of the brain through synaptic pruning (Santos, 2020). As soon as we reach ten years old, our brains have cut out as much as 50% of the synapses we had when we were only two years of age. This could be the reason why most of us have so few memories of our earliest years.

Let's take a look at some illustrations of brain plasticity at work so you can see that it is not just a wishful concept but can be applied to alter your brain for better use.

To become a taxi driver in London, one must pass the most difficult geography test in the world – the *Knowledge Test*. Memorizing it includes memorizing 20,000 landmarks, 320 main routes, and 25,000 streets. A research study conducted by neurologists of the University College of London discovered that an average cabbie develops a bigger hippocampus as a result of the memorization.

Some children are told by their parents, teachers, and fellow children that they aren't smart. This has an effect on the children and their future as this can become a self-fulfilling prophecy.

Carol Dweck, PhD., a world-renowned psychologist and professor of Stanford University discovered through her research study that when students are taught that intelligence is changeable, it made a significant effect on their morale and performance. It proves that by simply teaching them about brain plasticity and making them aware that they had the potential to get smarter and do better in school, their performance and confidence are enhanced (Bernard, 2010).

However, not all changes are positive, and like muscles, brain cells degenerate when not in use. There are areas in the brain that eventually get smaller when you aren't using them. So when you don't use certain neural connections, they too can wither and die. Also, not all neural connections are positive. Negative brain plasticity can cause destructive addictions, bad habits, and negative self-talk to be firmly entrenched and, therefore, hard to change.

Evidence showing negative brain plasticity is about animal domestication. Animals that are cared for as pets have smaller brain mass than animals living in the wilds (Weiner, 2017). Wolves have larger brains compared to dogs of the same body size.

People who are interested in the study of wolves discovered that they are smarter than domesticated dogs in every significant way. For while dogs living with human beings excel at reading humans, they don't have much use of their brainpower required for food hunting in the wilds. Their survival instinct is somehow lowered and the same thing holds true for us ("Who's (Socially) Smarter: The Dog or the Wolf?" 2017).

CREATE A BETTER BRAIN USING SELF-DIRECTED BRAIN PLASTICITY

Self-Directed Neuroplasticity refers to the process of intentionally utilizing your child's brain malleability to make your kids smarter. The brain will inevitably change so whether those changes are for better or worse, that is largely up to you. You can wait to see how your child's brain will develop or actively involve yourself in moving your child's brain in the direction you want. What is important is the fact that there are steps you can take to encourage brain plasticity for your children and keep their brain regrowing and reorganizing.

Now, let's take a look at some ways to do it and then you can find practical ways to use brain plasticity to improve your child's intelligence and cognitive functions.

Research proves that the brain never stops changing as long as your child continues learning new things. Consider the following activities in encouraging your children to explore and discover new things and ways:

Dancing can stimulate the release of Brain-Derived Neurotrophic Factor (BDNF) – a protein that helps develop growth, maintenance, and brain plasticity required for learning and memory (Hanna, 2017).

Music helps enhance attention, memory, neuroplasticity, and child's learning (Steele, 2013).

Arts improve fluid intelligence, Intelligence Quotient, attention, and neuroplasticity (Dana Foundation, 2010).

Studying new languages enlarges the language centers in the brain as well as the hippocampus.

Magnetic Resonance Imaging (MRI) results have proven that learning a new language develops a new level of connectivity ("Learning languages is a workout for brains, both young and old | Penn State University," 2014).

MIND MAPPING

Do you want your children to have better grades with less work?

It is normal for children to find class activities boring and tedious. However, there's a new way to make schoolwork fun and enjoyable for children. It is a secret formula that uses just a few colored pens and a brain-boosting activity.

A Mind Map is a quick, easy, and interesting way to receive, store, and use information.

Here is how Mind Mapping can be helpful to your children.

- It makes listening and taking notes easy and not boring
- It helps your child's studying and revising to be fast and effective
- It helps your child generate ideas or brainstorm for any project activity

A Mind Map incorporates words, pictures, and colors into the learning process which makes it a delightful way for children to explore, learn, and study. In short, Mind Mapping is a beneficial learning tool to help your children:

- Remember things better
- Generate new brilliant ideas
- Save time and be more productive
- Get higher grades
- Organize their thoughts and activities
- Find school learning more fun and exciting!

Let's get more specific to better understand what Mind Mapping is all about.

Mind Mapping And The Brain

It is common knowledge that our brain is divided into two hemispheres - the right hemisphere and the left hemisphere. The left side of the brain is associated with linear, logical, sequential, analytical, and objective reasoning while the right side is creative, intuitive, fantasy-oriented, visual, and holistic. Although children tend to lean on one side in how they think, they are more right-brained.

The way we raised our children and their surroundings determine if they end-up as a right or left thinker. With this in mind, by putting much effort into nurturing our children to utilize both sides of their brain, we can help them grow their potentials.

In one of the articles published in MY INK Blog entitled Left-Brain vs. Right-Brain, the author explained how *designers* and *developers* think.

According to the aforementioned article, the developer is inclined to use their left-brain while designers are more on their right-brain. Although both utilize the standard way of thinking which enables them to perform the necessary functions required for their job, it likewise creates limitations and oversights as they are not using both hemispheres of their brain.

To illustrate, let's understand that a designer focuses on color, branding, and aesthetics. Because they are more on visuals and creativity, they want their creation to be visually appealing. Therefore, it is usual for a designer to overlook other things like form testing and proper coding practices.

So, to help your children learn to use both sides of their brains, teaching them about the Mind Mapping Technique is the best way to do it. Mind mapping combines elements that appeal to both left and right side hemispheres and thus optimizes the brain's ability to create and learn.

To better understand how a Mind Map can help your children, here's how it works.

- There are five easy steps involved in mind mapping.

- Make sure to use blank sheets of paper that are not lined instead of the usually lined papers commonly used by children in school. Place the paper sideways.
- Using colored pens, draw a picture in the middle of the page of the topic you have in mind.
- Think of things to represent your main ideas about the topic and draw them surrounding the first picture you just made. Draw heavy connecting curved lines from the main picture (topic) to each of the pictures representing main ideas. Note that at this point, you are teaching your children to use both sides of the brain. Words are then underlined throughout the Mind Map as keywords.
- You can then think of other things (sub-ideas) to expand or support your main ideas and draw lines connecting sub-ideas to the main idea.

Your mind map should look like a tree with a main trunk and branches which can further have twigs (minor points).

TYPES OF INTELLIGENCE

A child's learning capability can be maximized if the learning style is suitable to his learning method preference. By learning style, we use this to describe how a child learns. Note that children differ in their learning preferences.

One child may learn best through visuals while another by movement, touch, hearing, etc. However, labeling children as having just one learning style could be incorrect and limiting the child's capability to learn more. The truth is, children, learn in a variety of ways. While a child may absorb information through visuals at one time, he may able to learn something more through movement in another situation.

To better understand the individuality of learning, let us first understand the theory of Multiple Intelligences as defined by Howard Gardner, Professor of Cognition and Education at Harvard Graduate School of Education.

Gardner's theory of Multiple Intelligences disputes the idea that we are born with a single intelligence that can be measured through IQ tests, and that this intelligence can't be changed. The traditional theory of intelligence created a mindset that a person can either be smart or not based on their IQ test result.

According to Gardner's theory, there are at least eight different intelligences and all human beings are born with all of these Multiple Intelligences.

Furthermore, Gardner asserts that each individual has unique and distinct intelligence profiles as shaped by their genes and surroundings. Therefore, one child may have a strong musical intelligence while another child may have a strong inclination towards linguistic intelligence.

Here are the different types of Multiple Intelligence as described in the theory developed by Dr. Gardner.

Visual-Spatial Intelligence

This refers to the ability to visualize and create something in a space, such as what engineers, architects, designers, and artists do. Those who excel in this type of intelligence have the following abilities:

- Mental Imagery
- Visual Manipulation
- Spatial Reasoning
- Artistic skills

Logical-Mathematical

This refers to the logical and mathematical abilities. It is characterized by deductive and inductive reasoning associated with an individual's understanding of concepts and abstract ideas. Also, this helps them effortlessly identify patterns, codes, sequences, and relationships. The learning style for those with this type of intelligence involves obtaining abstract knowledge of concepts before they can work on the details.

Those with logical-mathematical intelligence have the following characteristics:

- Enjoy games that focus on logic and strategy
- Fond of conducting investigations and experiments to prove hypotheses
- Good in different tasks that involve numbers and quantifying things (e.g. arithmetic problems and mathematical operations)
- Enjoy solving puzzles and mysteries

Linguistic Intelligence

This type of intelligence refers to a person's ability to learn languages and dialects as well as communicate effectively – using the right words to express and influence others.

Children with linguistic intelligence have the following characteristics:

- Enjoy reading and writing
- Good in remembering written and verbal information
- Enjoy word games, crossword puzzles, and other similar games
- Frequently use humor in telling stories
- Effectively use words to persuade, inspire, and influence others to accomplish a purpose
- Easily learn languages and dialects

Musical Intelligence

Children with this type of intelligence are sensitive to sounds and can distinguish tones, rhythm, timbre, and pitch. They are aware even of sounds that aren't noticeable to others and can connect emotions with music. Children who are musically inclined can identify, create, reproduce, understand, and translate music. Musically inclined children:

- Love music
- Easily memorize songs and melodies
- Extremely sensitive to sounds and their patterns
- Enjoy singing and/or playing musical instruments
- Easily discern, identify, and categorize sounds
- Can create, reflect on, and express themselves through music

Bodily-Kinesthetic Intelligence

Children with this type of intelligence have developed physical control and motor skills. They exhibit a high level of hand-eye coordination as that of the body and mind. The athletic types often have these capabilities but it is rarely recognized as intelligence. Have you ever heard an athlete being recognized as intelligent because of his athletic skills?

Those who have bodily-kinesthetic intelligence display the following characteristics:

- Love to do or create something with their hands
- They are aware of their physical capabilities and limitations
- They have no issues with touching or being touched by others
- They can handle tools and equipment with precision and accuracy.
- Effectively communicate well using gestures, actions, and body language

Interpersonal Intelligence

It is the ability to understand other people and know how to effectively interact with them based on that understanding. This social skill includes the capability to identify distinctions among people, sensitivity to the temperaments and moods of other people, and perform effective verbal and nonverbal communication.

Individuals who have a high level of interpersonal intelligence have a high emotional quotient which makes them good potential leaders or great leaders.

Children with interpersonal intelligence possess the following characteristics:

- Easily identify a specific person even amongst the crowd
- See and understand situations, opinions, and ideas from various perspectives instead of merely sticking to their line of thinking

- Are extroverts; they feel recharged being with people
- Easily distinguish differences and distinctions among people
- Have a wide circle of acquaintances and friends
- Good knack at resolving conflict and maintaining peace in groups

Intra-Personal Intelligence

Awareness of oneself is another type of intelligence. Knowing and understanding who you are and how you feel is an indication that you have intra-personal intelligence.

This type of intelligence also shows respect and appreciation for the human condition.

Children with intra-personal intelligence possess these characteristics:

- Independent and strong-willed
- Can motivate themselves
- Have a high level of self-awareness and clearly understand what they want and what they have
- Tend to put themselves first when assessing different situations
- Are introverts and prefer to be alone by themselves to enjoy peace
- Can generate own ideas and implement actions out of those ideas without leaning on others
- Enjoys reading and exploring things

Naturalist Intelligence

A child with this intelligence loves and understands

nature. They are sensitive to the natural world and love to contribute to its development.

Children who are born naturalists:

- Love nature itself and learning things concerning it
- Love nurturing the environment and discovering new species
- Enjoy spending time and exploring outdoors (e.g. hiking, gardening, and camping)
- Can easily establish a connection with animals
- Talented in raising animals and plants
- Interested in various natural science subjects like botany, zoology, meteorology, and biology
- Can easily find patterns and relationships to nature

Existential Intelligence

This intelligence involves sensitivity, awareness, and concern with the ultimate sense of being. Characteristics of those with existential intelligence include:

- Exhibiting a high level of sensitivity in matters in connection with human existence
- Having a genuine curiosity and are not afraid to ask questions like, "What's my purpose of living?", "Is there life after death?" or "Does God truly exist?"

CHAPTER 2

LEARNING STYLES

LEARNING styles group common ways that children use to learn and every child has a mixture of different learning styles. Some children have a dominant style of learning and use less of the other learning styles. Others use different styles in different situations. There is no right combination, neither is there a fixed one.

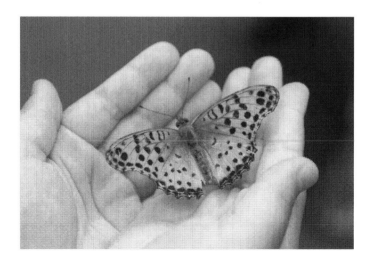

Your child can always develop their abilities in less dominant styles or further develop styles that are already used well.

Your child's method of learning is determined by their representational systems (or learning styles). Some children gather more learning information through their eyes (**Visual**) while others get it through physical exercises (**Kinesthetic**). Still, others gather information through variable tones and in entertaining ways (**Auditory**).

Combining learning styles and multiple intelligences for learning is relatively a new approach that educators are just starting to recognize. The traditional way of teaching that many continue to use is mainly linguistic and logical. Many of our educators are still using a limited range of learning and teaching techniques. They still rely on classroom and book-based learning where many repetitions and tests actually subject children to pressures.

But because of the so-called *Digital Age,* more children learn to process thoughts and think at the same time, making them *Auditory Digital*. However, most schools fail to recognize this, eventually leading to children encountering difficulties in learning. Instead of teaching them how to understand, they are taught how to listen, read and repeat the entire lecture daily.

Not all children process information in the same way. Needless to say, our learning styles vary with each other. According to the studies of Neuro-Linguistic Programming, there are four known learning styles, which can be also called *representational systems* or *modalities*. These are the styles used by different people to process and share information as well as representing the world through our senses.

WHY SOME CHILDREN FAIL?

Just like in adults, children gather and learn information differently. *Visual children* prefer to learn through images or pictures. *Auditory children* learn through conversational methods. *Kinesthetic children* collect information and learn through physical exercises or activities while the *Auditory Digital* types learn mainly through listening and taking notes.

Because of this, the existing educational system considers Auditory Digital types as smart or bright. In other words, if the students are visual types and teachers fail to show them diagrams and pictures, it is more likely for these children to fail even when these children are studying inside a private school. If the teacher fails to adjust their teaching to following the children's learning style, they will be at a disadvantage. In the end, the children will just stay ignorant, regardless of how much time and effort the teacher spent in teaching them.

Through the use of perception, which happens when our brain receives certain information as well as its meaning, this can help determine a person's learning style, especially children. Even if everyone can use all of the learning styles, the truth remains that there's a particular style that we prefer or favor over the others.

According to suggested statistics in most developed countries (St. Louis, 2020),

- 65% of the people are Visual
- 30% percent are Auditory
- 5% percent are Kinesthetic

Visual learner

Visual children do more things quickly. They can describe a picture more quickly than other learners and often use gestures. They are also conscious of their appearance and tend to be neat and well-organized.

Because visual learners focus on images, they find it hard to remember instructions because their mind is busy exploring through a collage of mental images and they describe situations as seen in photographs. Visual children's handwriting is almost incorrigible because they tend to write quickly.

Auditory Learner

Auditory learners are sensitive to voices and sounds, and they rhythmically do things. If you see children who read with their lips, they are most likely to be auditory learners. They also love to engage in monologue or self-talk. However, when others make a noise, they find it annoying.

Children with the auditory learning preference process information through hearing and they benefit most from oral instruction. They also enjoy listening to music and are those children who can easily memorize rhymes and songs.

Kinesthetic Learner

In contrast to visual learners, kinesthetic learners do things more slowly and when they speak, there is that long pause in between statements as they love to feel whatever information is fed to them and process it accurately.

They likewise respond best to physical regards, including touching. So, when teaching them, it is recommended to give them a mild touch or a brief pat in the shoulder to have their full attention.

Children like these tend to move closer to the one teaching them and are more comfortable with hand gestures compared to other learners of different learning style preferences. They also have this tendency to feel one's energy and can relate to their emotions more effectively.

Auditory-Digital Learner

Auditory-digital learners tend to exhibit a combination of these learning styles characteristics.

Before giving their answer to a question, they are repeating it in their heads which is why they take a longer time to process information and answer the question. Needless to say, they are the ones you can't rush.

While visual learners learn to collect information via images, auditory-digital learners give more value on logic and details. They have this tendency to use acronyms, jargon, and symbolism when giving examples. They lean more on the intellectual side and their feelings are more attached to words rather than to results.

They are not easy to convince unless you have proof.

YOUR CHILD'S LEARNING STRENGTHS

Based on your child's learning style preference, you can identify where your child belongs under the two learning strength categories to put their learning capability to optimal use.

. . .

LEARNING-STRENGTH CATEGORIES

We have identified two learning-strength categories.

- Visual-Spatial-Kinesthetic (VSK)
- Auditory-Sequential (AS)

Notice that these two learning-strength categories are a fusion of your child's dominant intelligence based on Multiple Intelligence Theory and learning style preferences.

As soon as you identify your child's learning-strength, you can find learning ways and strategies suitable to it and thus can maximize their learning experiences and put them to optimal use.

As a way of knowing your child's learning-strength, consider their learning experiences and determine which among these are first most enjoyable, and then most frustrating. Does your child connect more to what he or she sees, hears, or feels? When bringing them to the zoo, do they easily connect with their favorite animal's habitat and excitedly describe to you what they feel or see?

By observing your child's likes and dislikes, you can easily discover their learning preferences and intelligence. Note that your child's world is a mixture of multiple intelligence and learning styles, so don't confine them to only one of these.

VISUAL-SPATIAL-KINESTHETIC (VSK)

Children with VSK strength are said to be sensitive to physical, spatial, and temporal relationships of ideas, objects, or images in and through space and time. Children working under this type of learning-strength are good at mentally recreating and visualizing spatial relationships. They are also seeing the big picture instead of concentrating only on a certain aspect. Children with VSK have this ability to predict sequence, fine coordination, and motor skills. Also, they are good in the visualization of movements, physical coordination, and a time-coordination sense that give them the ability to easily put together broken objects or puzzles.

If your child is a VSK learner, they can easily:

- Respond to an idea being introduced before details are covered.
- Explore the big picture or concept before getting into smaller details
- Discover and create relationships between themselves and things they are about to learn
- Explain and make demonstrations of images, visuals, videos, diagrams, maps, charts, photos, and anything with graphics
- Learn with own diagrams, maps, or arts
- Visualize patterns and connections and learn through video, books with diagrams and pictures, and other visual memory strategies
- Create analogies for strong relational-memory building
- Use movements of their bodies or other objects to learn information, convey ideas and solve problems
- Spot opportunities to discover new things and ways to solve problems, and analyze them, based on their intuition and reasoning
- Establish hands-on experiments and manipulate objects to deduce patterns

- Good in dramatization, puppet shows, and pantomimes
- Make crafts, puzzles, models, and manipulate blocks and Lego pieces
- Move letters on magnetic boards, prefer typing over handwriting, and when writing, they are more comfortable writing on blackboards or whiteboards than on papers
- Step on number lines
- Love and enjoy nature walks and field trips

VSK children likewise face many challenges.

- They have trouble organizing time and prioritizing activities
- They easily get distracted or tune out in passive learning, prolonged sitting, and extended explanations
- They experience difficulty with verbally communicating their visualization or concepts
- They feel more challenged by memorization and are able to write down all the steps they are thinking when solving problems compared to linguistic learners

Auditory-Sequential (AS)

Children with Auditory-Sequential strength exhibit sensitivity to words, sounds, logic, structured patterns, order, and sequence. Their proficiencies may include many of the following: logical deduction, concept-building, and organizational abilities.

Children that are Auditory-Sequential are analytical learners and they tend to process information in parts to the whole manner, as opposed to VK learners. AS learners respond to logic, order, and sequence. Preference of this learning style is evident in children who respond best to spoken information. These children often have linguistic and logical-mathematical intelligence strengths and they tend to learn best by evaluating patterns and connections in the information they hear.

AS children also respond well when studying information methodically as in lists, timelines, and other sequences using information they need to learn. They also respond well to reading aloud to themselves, talking, or being verbally tested when studying.

AS learners tend to be analytical, they prefer dealing with one task at a time in an organized working space. They also prefer solving existing issues, rather than develop their own, and they use logic and deduction when solving these issues.

If your child happens to be an AS learner, you will see that they enjoy expanding their own concept or idea by reasoning out and predicting logical implications that follow a certain rule or guiding principle. They, likewise, prefer learning activities that have one correct answer that can be broken down into logical, sequential steps.

AS learners easily respond to:

- Clear rules to follow in learning a skill or in doing an activity or structured sequential notes
- Categorization and assortments
- Existing problems
- One task at a time
- Memorizing facts presented in logical and methodological order

- Written and spoken language (including tone, rhythm, and pitch changes)
- Songs and music, audiobooks – connecting music and rhythm to learning
- Reading aloud and repeating information to themselves when studying

CHAPTER 3

THE IMPORTANCE OF READING

WHEN YOUR CHILD starts learning to read, they are starting to recognize similarities and differences in letters. You can help boost their learning progress by encouraging them to recognize word patterns. Through this, you would be helping your child discover gradually through many challenges.

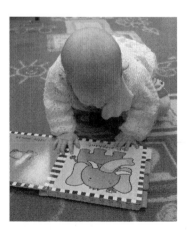

Reading is an essential part of learning. To some children, reading can come easily, but to others, it can be a struggle. There are some complex processes involved in reading that makes these children struggle as in:

- Recognizing words
- Sounding out words with different pronunciations
- Fluent reading with expressiveness
- Memorizing high-sounding vocabulary
- Reading comprehension
- Understanding vocabulary

All these lead to a discouraging learning environment for struggling children.

Learning to read must not evoke this kind of emotion in children for when they experience negative emotions or pressures, your child will have a hard time learning. Instead of developing their ability to learn, it will be hampered and affect other areas of learning development as well. When learning to read becomes frustrating for these children they stop caring about books completely. If learning to read is hard, they would rather opt for some other means like watching television or playing video games. Learning to read must not be a joyless struggle for your child.

Pattern Identification Activities

The brain identifies and keeps information by recognizing certain patterns. A child is learning when his brain recognizes something new that fits into a familiar pattern. It provides the association with the new sensory information and stores it into the memory circuit.

It is normal for children during their first and second

years to get confused with numbers and letters. However, if you noticed that your child commits more mistakes than normal while trying to associate a certain letter with the wrong sound, or distinguishing words that rhyme, then you should have your child assessed by a specialist. If intervention is needed, then it can be given as early as possible.

Here are activities you can do with your child to help them improve.

Words That Sounds Alike

Introduce to them words that end with the same sound.

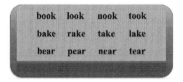

When reading with your child, try changing your vocal pitch, tone, speed, and volume to emphasize words with the same sound for auditory patterns.

Say a series of words with the same beginning or ending sounds.

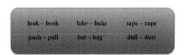

Words with the Same Meaning

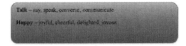

Matching Words with Images

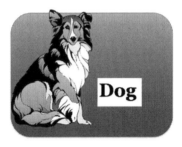

WORD GAMES

Here are games you may use to help your children practice word patterns - spelling recognition and patterns, as well as letter-sound knowledge. When using any of these games, choose words from books you are reading with your child. These games are designed to promote a strong sense of competence and success in a child.

CONCENTRATION

- Choose 5-10 words from a book you recently read with your child.
- One by one, print them in bold letters on a 3x5-inch index card. Make a pair of each word or give your child an index card and let them copy the word you wrote on the card.

- Shuffle cards and lay them face down in a row. Take two cards and read the words. If the two cards match, keep them and get another two cards. If the cards don't match, let your child take his/her turn to repeat what you have done. Play until all the cards are taken. The one with the most number of cards is the winner.

The purpose of this game exercise is to develop your child's ability to recognize words. If they have trouble recognizing the word, say it and let your child sound it out. Depending on the age of your child, you can control the difficulty of the game by the choice of words or the number of words used.

For very early learners, choose words that are easy to distinguish visually like "mother", "sun", or "dark." To make it more challenging for your child, also include words that aren't commonly distinctive like, "this and that" "when, where, and what."

Variation:
You may use a rhyming pair of words like...

- bark - park
- nook - look
- make - bake
- hair - pair

Another variation of this game is letter-sound recognition.

- D - dog
- C - cat
- B - bird

For older children, you may introduce a variation that includes vocabulary exercises using homonyms (words that sound alike but with different spelling and meaning).

Example:

- There - their
- Hear - here
- Sea – See

BUTTON MATCHING ACTIVITY

Collect buttons and group them according to color, number of holes, design, and shape. Allow your child to add buttons to each group and see if they can recognize patterns. Ask them why they choose certain buttons to be included in the group of buttons.

Add more complex patterns by providing a selection of single-colored against multi-colored buttons or metal buttons vs. plastic buttons. However, be aware that buttons and other small objects can pose hazards to little children. They have a tendency to put little things in their mouths because of curiosity and can choke in the process. You may also use other objects like Lego toy components and other materials. There is no limit to the materials you may use.

WHAT BELONGS – WHAT DOESN'T BELONG

This activity will challenge and build more connections to the way letters and words form patterns.

Directions:

Choose three items with the same characteristics. Let your child find what these things have in common.

Group another three items. Two of these items have

something in common but the other one is different. Let your child point out which one is different and must not belong to the group. Let them explain why they should not be in that group.

As your child begins to master the difference, create more complex groupings like using money of different values. For example, sort coins into pennies, nickels, and dimes. Later, you can level up to pattern sequencing.

Here are some examples:

- Penny-penny-dime
- Penny-dime-dime
- Penny-nickel-dime

Allow your child to add coins following the same pattern. This will build in your child the patterning skills for reading and sequencing skills for numeracy – the basics of mathematical learning.

VISUALIZING PATTERN AND ACTIVE LISTENING

To help your children build up their vocabulary and remember the meaning of words, adopt the visualization technique. The more your child uses creativity and energy in visualizing, the stronger the neural network he builds will be.

There are two different ways to make the visualization more effective. One is by hearing while reading and another is by verbally summarizing what they had just read. Children can directly visualize things they hear or see and even more when these are incorporated with color, movement, and object manipulation.

CHAPTER 4

THE IMPORTANCE OF MATH

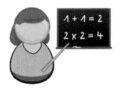

Math is associated with the fields of science, technology, and engineering. However, math goes beyond mere numbers, formulas, or equations. It develops skills and analytical thinking required to help children master various disciplines. That is to say, math isn't just the foundation for careers in science but of every aspect of learning.

Parents who want to predict their child's progress can gauge it through the child's mathematical skills. In a 2007 study conducted with 35,000 preschoolers across England, Canada, and the US, researchers found that early math skills can be the strongest determiner for later success (Leopold, 2007).

Children who excel in math also stand out in reading, writing, and communicating. Learning mathematics can benefit children in more ways than we commonly anticipate. It helps children develop their confidence and helps form the basic foundation for many aspects of our daily life.

Learning math also supports children's literacy development. Children who can communicate effectively can master math with their mathematical understanding and enhance their linguistic fluency such as vocabulary, grammar, oral language abilities, and comprehension. Thus, if you expose your child to math at a young age, there's a better chance for them to excel in language too.

MATHEMATICAL READINESS

Math exposure is closely associated with elementary and later school success. Children with a strong foundation of basic math skills such as naming numbers, counting, and ordering conditions are able to master math and problem solving much better as they grow up.

To ensure that your child isn't left behind, you need to train them to attain the level of competent understanding at a young age. Exposed below are two major pointers on how you can do it.

EXPOSE YOUR CHILD TO MATHEMATICAL CONCEPTS

Mathematical concepts are established in a logical and gradual progression. When your child is forced to learn addition and multiplication even before they understand the relationships between quantities and numerals, they will only end up memorizing mathematical facts.

However, when they are trained with the activities according to their abilities and developmental level, there will be a natural progression from one level to another. They will mentally prosper in culturally meaningful and linguistically abundant mathematical activities.

PROVIDE YOUR CHILD WITH THE RIGHT SUPPORT

As a parent, you are the best person who can offer your child the best support for their learning and advancement. If you want your child to flourish, put them in rich learning environments that can stimulate their brain better. Your proper guidance and feedback also make a great difference in their development. You can also get supplemental support from excellent early math programs as well as highly motivated teachers or tutors.

Activities such as baking, planning a simple party, integrating math into your bedtime stories, and playing Legos together can be enjoyable learning opportunities for your child. Take these simple bonding moments to have fun with your children and encourage them to develop their math skills at the same time.

THE IMPORTANCE OF MATH AT AN EARLY AGE

Math is an integral part of learning for every child in their early years. Receiving a well-rounded foundation in math is an essential life skill. Numeracy is the ability to apply math concepts in all areas of life. Perceiving and using shapes and measurements can develop their spatial abilities. Recognizing, describing, and creating described patterns are essential factors that can help a child's problem-solving skills.

When you introduce math to your child from an early age, they develop their understanding of all problem-solving elements and deepen their reasoning abilities of distinct concepts.

Every child can be successful with math, provided that they're allowed to understand it through the most practical method for them. Parents should ensure that their children are motivated, engaged, and can implement critical thinking since these are key requirements for math.

Even at infancy, babies are known to have the ability to display essential mathematical abilities. For instance, they can identify various sets of objects with different quantities, or they can find objects in a specified location. It doesn't take a mathematical whiz of a parent to integrate math into your child's daily life.

Infant To Toddler

There are a lot of ways on how you can introduce math to your infant or toddler. You can present numbers and counting by reading storybooks or looking out for shapes in a game. Let me provide you some examples:

Teach them how to count through visual aids. Your child can respond better when you introduce numbers and counting with the help of the objects they see. However, remember that one child differs from another. What may work for one may not work for others.

Use familiar objects. You don't have to purchase learning tools every single time. As a matter of fact, familiar objects such as money, trees, pens, candies, and household things are good enough to help them.

Use games. Playing math games teaches your child that learning math is an enjoyable process. This doesn't limit them to Sudoku, Monopoly or other similar games. You can be as creative as you can since the most fun games come from your own imagination.

Integrate math into your everyday life. It can be counting how many cars you see on the road or how much money do you need to buy ten pieces of candy. You can give them simple math problems and guide them as they look for the right answers.

The key is to make learning math enjoyable. Learning math isn't limited to the classroom-type of learning. That can be tedious and boring for an infant or toddler. In effect, they will easily associate math as a hard and frustrating experience.

PRESCHOOLER

Most preschoolers are interested in math even if they still don't know that what they're actually curious about is "math." They're in the stage where they are fascinated by a lot of things. The best way for parents to cultivate their preschoolers' interest in math is to engage their children in dynamic, hands-on games and activities.

Preschoolers love to ask questions and do activities that involve various aspects of math. Even though they may not have memorized numbers yet, they will begin to understand the mathematical concept.

PRIMARY SCHOOL LEVEL

As a parent, you're the best example for your child. Show them that you value and acknowledge their achievement to motivate them further. Help them develop an attitude that being good at math isn't all about being inherently smart, but by consistently working on their skills.

In a study conducted by the University of Missouri in the USA, it was revealed that children who do not understand the meaning and function of numbers before entering the first grade have slower progress compared to those who learned it. A higher percentage of these children cannot catch up and, therefore, have heightened risk for low scores in math through the seventh grade.

Remember, all children have the potential to learn and excel in math. All you need to do is to give them the opportunity to enhance this potential and support them throughout their developmental stage.

STRATEGIES & ACTIVITIES TO ENHANCE YOUR CHILD'S MATHEMATICAL PROWESS

We may not love math, but that doesn't mean that our children should share the same distaste for the subject. After all, it's one of the most important subjects our children will learn in school. Let me show you some essential tips that can help you boost your child's mathematical prowess.

Set Your Biases Aside

You may not have a great experience with math during your childhood, but that shouldn't mean that your child would undergo the same process. Allow your child to start in a clean slate; meaning, don't introduce any biases or fears to your child about math. Let them discover how exciting and incredible the subject can be.

Don't Introduce Math As A Hard Subject

Again, don't let your child think that math is only for geniuses or for those whose genetic make-up allows them to excel in the subject. Every child has the potential to be a mathematical expert. Your fear or bias can only have a negative influence on your child. Avoid instilling in your child's mind that math is a difficult subject. Always take a positive route to help your child progress and be an achiever. This is true not only about learning math but also about other subjects or aspects of life.

Start Early

Train your child while it's still early so that they can naturally accept it as part of their daily life. When you integrate learning the mathematical concepts into their everyday routine, you also bring them towards excellence in the subject.

Start teaching them while they're still infants. The beauty of the internet era is that you can easily access information to help you gain ideas on how you can hone your child's math skills. You can train them to spot patterns and shapes in an interesting way. You can introduce numbers to them since these are basic and easy to understand.

Focus On The Process

As grown-ups, we tend to focus on a result-oriented approach to learning. However, this shouldn't be the case for children who are still starting to learn about concepts. It's okay for them not to get the answers correctly the first time. It's normal for them to make mistakes from time-to-time because, through these, they learn better and experience progress.

Be patient in showing them the right process on how they can come up with the right answer on their own effort. Don't rush because your child can pick up their speed later on. More importantly, don't stress them out just because you're getting impatient. Stress can demotivate them and instill fear instead of confidence.

. . .

Help Them Understand The Relevance Of Math

One of the best ways to motivate a child in learning math is to help them understand its relevance in the real world. Teach them that the knowledge they are acquiring today will be useful as they get older. Provide them an example, such as the importance of counting money or how proper measurements of food ingredients can affect the taste of food. Give them a real talk on how math works in our day-to-day lives.

Teach Math Progressively

The structure of your math "lessons" greatly affects your child's performance. Make it progressive; which means that you need to start with the most basic. From the foundational concepts, the lessons should progress in difficulty. After all, it doesn't make sense when you teach them multiplication right away without teaching them addition before that.

Gearing up your child to excel in math shouldn't be too difficult. You have the right resources and can seek various ways to make it fun and enjoyable, not only for your child but also for you.

CHAPTER 5

ENHANCE YOUR CHILD IQ

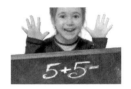

HOW IS IQ MEASURED?

INTELLIGENCE QUOTIENT or IQ is a measure of your child's reasoning ability which is a relationship between their potential and the normal statistics of all possible results.

To determine your child's IQ, they are tested based on concrete and abstract reasoning based on their age and development norms.

Measuring IQ involves a series of tasks measuring different measures of intelligence including

- Short-term memory
- Spatial recognition
- Mathematical ability
- Analytical thinking

Note that the IQ test is not designed to measure the amount of information one has learned but their capacity to learn.

BUILDING UPON INTELLIGENCE

There are many ways to build up your child's intelligence and IQ. According to a study conducted by Stanford University School of Medicine, personalized tutoring, when coupled with mathematical learning, can improve children's memory. It likewise suggests that when a child can solve basic arithmetic problems from memory, they can also handle more complex problems.

Provide Your Child With The Right Foundation

To make sure that you are building the right foundation for your child, use an approach that blends the benefits of personalized teaching with the discipline of self-learning and self-discovery. Such an approach is designed to introduce your child to new concepts in incremental steps that will make learning math easier for your child.

On top of personalized training, it is through the different brain functions – brainstorming, understanding ideas, critical thinking, and logical reasoning along with practice that improves and deepens your child's understanding. Practice alone is not enough to make your child understand concepts.

So, if your child garners a low IQ score, it doesn't mean that it can't be changed. Encouraging them to indulge in problem-solving, logical, and critical thinking will provide them the opportunities to do better in the future. What is important is the fact that IQ can be changed and all you need is to exercise your child's brain through early exposure to Mathematics.

.   .   .

Read To Your Child

Reading with your child is significant to linguistic learning, or the ability to process information with the use of words and language. It is more challenging compared to processing images or speech as parts of the brain are making connections.

As your child reads, it helps improve their language which is essential for communication and everyday tasks. Reading not only helps improve language but also keeps their mind sharp. Helping your child to read early may not only help the growth of your child's literacy but also benefit your child's wider range of cognitive abilities, crucial to them in later life.

Early reading is also important in predicting a lifetime of literacy experience. A study made by Professors, Anne E. Cunningham and Keith E. Stanovich, disclosed that students who learned to read early are more likely to read more. The study stated further that reading volume had a significant contribution to vocabulary, spelling, and verbal fluency (Cunningham & Stanovich, 1998). In simple words, reading can make your child grow smarter. As your child grows older, introduce concept stories to help expand their vocabulary and visualization for them to have a better understanding of abstract concepts.

Introduce Child To Spatial Intelligence-Building Activities

Allow your child to play with memory games, puzzles, mazes, crafts, and toy figurines as these tools help build their spatial intelligence. Playing with blocks and construction is particularly significant and beneficial to your child as it gives them opportunities for multiple learning.

While engaging in games that involve structures and blocks, children develop their spatial awareness and spatial intelligence. Spatial intelligence is the ability to visualize. Stacking blocks will allow your child to use their spatial intelligence. Developing spatial skills likewise supports your child's learning in areas of Science, Technology, Engineering, and Mathematics.

An early introduction to visualization and spatial relationships were found to develop stronger Arithmetic skills in primary learners.

Let Your Child Do Math And Physical Exercises To Develop Fluid Intelligence

Fluid intelligence is the ability to think in an abstract dimension, solve problems, identify patterns, and discern relationships even without the use of prior knowledge. Fluid intelligence is used when exposed to new situations.

You can help your child gain this ability by teaching them the relationship between objects using concrete examples. For example, to teach your child the different shapes, you have to show them objects in varying shapes so they can see the real differences. Allow them to touch and feel objects while comparing them. When teaching about numbers and quantity, use objects for them to see. Let's say you are introducing 1, 2, and 3. You may use 1 ball, 2 balls, and 3 balls for them to identify the difference in numbers.

Besides exposing your child early to Mathematics, learning physical exercises can likewise develop fluid intelligence. It is said that certain hormones are released when doing physical activities and such hormones are beneficial to the hippocampus, or that portion of the brain associated with learning and memory.

Therefore, let your child run, play, and tumble as long as you are there to see that they are safe!

Have Confidence In Your Children

Regardless of your child's abilities and intelligence, be there for them! It matters greatly to support your child with praises and rewards every time they try doing well on something to boost their confidence.

A study on a group of students randomly selected proved that students who were told by their teacher that they are SMART showed a higher average IQ score compared to the rest of the students although there were no special tests done to single out these students who were selected at random. This proves that whatever you say to your child can have an impact on their learning process.

Praise Their Efforts

Praising your child's efforts can have an impact on their performance and helps them develop a growth mindset.

Praise is most effective when focused on your child's effort and commitment and not on the result. Note that the emphasis of your praise should be to focus on their effort regardless of the result of their performance.

A Stanford University professor, Carol Dweck came up with Growth Mindset and Fixed Mindset concepts. According to her, Fixed Mindset concept states that intelligence is a fixed trait and nothing can be done to change this. On the other hand, Growth Mindset believes that intelligence and abilities are continuously developed throughout a person's life (Dweck, 2007, pp. 1–3).

THINGS TO DO AT HOME TO ENHANCE YOUR CHILD'S IQ

We can enhance our child's IQ by creating a highly conducive environment for both emotional and cognitive growth. By surrounding children with books and educational toys, these things will leave positive imprints in their brain, which will be brought along in their teenage years.

Streamlining and organizing your child's thought process to match a stimulating setting is required in improving your child's intelligence. Through conducting mathematics and unstructured play activities, your child will develop their fluid intelligence, and capacity to learn, as well as sharpen their creativity.

Listed below are some of the most widely-used ideas in creating a stimulating home for children's IQ:

Reinventing everyday objects. There is no definite or correct way of using or playing with objects when it comes to a child's imagination. Needless to say, a simple cardboard box that is used mainly for storing things can be a castle or fort while a plastic bottle can be a rocket ship or a submarine to a toddler. Finding creative uses for everyday things and objects allows children to stimulate their brain growth and become more flexible by using their imaginative capabilities. This also teaches them to engage and interact with people without preconceptions.

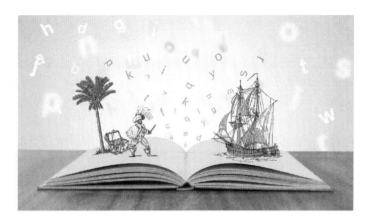

Introducing mathematics to them through stories

Research studies show that children are more likely to remember numbers, words, and events through hand gestures. So whenever you tell your child a story, don't forget to use gestures while encouraging them to follow suit. By mimicking actions, children learn techniques such as anticipation, evaluation, analysis, and facial recognition.

The simplest and yet the most effective way to pique a child's interest in math is through the use of picture books. Picture books are great tools to help young children learn language and math concepts.

Creating a construction or art corner at home

Set aside an area or room inside your home where your children can practice their art and building skills such as painting, clay sculpture, drawing, and much more. You can also set aside a part of their room for such a purpose, well-stocked with art and construction materials such as children's building blocks, clay, paper, paint, coloring pencils, and crayons.

The purpose is to provide your child with a personal space where they can make things and become messy according to their creativity. By letting them have time to create or play freely, you can help them develop their brains more. Through activities like molding, building, painting, drawing, and coloring, children exercise and train their creativity, imagination, and spatial skills, which rely on neural networks partially linked with mathematics.

Include mathematics in your conversations

By demonstrating the concept of numbers to your children, not only will they train their cognitive skills; it also builds their language communication and problem-solving skills. According to psychologist John Protzko, children that get exposed early to educational resources tend to gain a higher level of IQ compared to their peers who don't. The idea being taught here is to make them realize that math and learning, in general, are both memorable and fun. By using a good math program, children can engage with dialogue, games, props, and probing questions as well as a healthy dose of encouragement.

By simply saying statements such as "The food will be ready in ten minutes", "It will take an hour's drive to your grandparents' house", or "I gave you a bar of chocolate earlier. I'm giving you another two bars so that makes three", you are introducing numbers and math to your children in a simple yet fun and memorable way.

The simplest and yet the most effective way to pique a child's interest in math is through the use of picture books.

Picture books are great tools to help young children learn language and math concepts.

CHAPTER 6

BRAIN DEVELOPMENT DELAY

When there is a delay in the development of your child's brain to form long-term memories, including arithmetic facts such as multiplication tables, it does not mean that they won't be able to understand the concept of division in Mathematics. For children with delays in either short-term or long-term memory development, they can be equipped with a calculator to help them in their calculations so to progress with the other children in their class.

It can be frustrating for a child, and this is what usually holds them back to do basic arithmetic when they are learning mathematical operations. So while a child is still memorizing rote facts and they're actually supposed to learn new ideas, it will limit his understanding of the new lesson.

If your child has a learning problem, a calculator can address their delay issue especially when they are good at problem-solving and reasoning or logic but held back by errors in computation.

The best teachers continuously monitor a child's development levels and arrange them in groups where they are suited.

SHORT-TERM MEMORY PROBLEMS

The problem that children face in long-term memory is not storage but the capacity of the brain to retrieve stored information in long-term memory. An example of this is during an examination. Before they can answer a question, they need to retrieve information previously-stored so that they can give their answer.

To improve your child's long-term memory, make sure that they got enough sleep. Children who don't have enough sleep were shown to perform poorly on memory and attention tests.

Another way to train your child's long-term memory is to use predetermined sequences. For example, give them things to memorize like:

- 5 days of the week (Sunday, Monday, Tuesday ...)
- 12 months of the year (January, February, March ...)
- 9 Planets (Mercury, Venus, Earth . . .)
- NATO Phonetic Alphabet (Alpha, Bravo, Charlie ...)

IMPORTANT QUALITIES EVERY CHILD NEEDS

Intelligence Quotient can be a strong determinant of a child's performance in life as well as success. Here are some qualities that every child needs and which complement IQ.

Love Of Learning

Although a child may not be aware of it, they have a

positive attitude towards learning which plays a huge part of their future success. They start exploring their bodies at an early age and experiment with their different senses - see, hear, feel, taste, and touch.

Here are ways you can help to enhance their love for learning:

- Support their interest
- Make learning relevant to their everyday life
- Never discourage them with their ideas
- Support, accept, and inspire - while serving as a good model for them.

Motivation

Studies proved that effective studying techniques and those who are self-motivated develop the most improved Math skills. For parents to help motivate their children, addressing the following needs can help build a child's intrinsic motivation.

Autonomy

Children who feel they are being restrained lose their sense of motivation. Although we can't provide our children with total freedom, we can still provide them with other options. However, limit your option to two or three. It also helps to explain to your child why you can't permit them to do things they want.

Competence

When a child has failed in some activities, they have this tendency to feel embarrassed and avoid it. To prevent your child from experiencing this, praise them on how they tried their best and not on the outcome of their effort.

Develop in them the growth mindset while emphasizing that you are happy with their effort and they can do it better next time!

Connection

Children are best motivated when the source of motivation is related to them - their parents and peers. Remember that being fairly judged by an adult or having a feeling of being left out brings a negative emotion which can have a great impact on your child's learning.

Be a role model and always exercise patience and reasonable expectations while showering your child with encouragement. Your child may surprise you!

CHAPTER 7

MEMORY-ENHANCING LIFESTYLE

THE FIRST 1000 days in a human's life are vital to brain development. The way brain structure is developed during pregnancy, and in the first two years, constitutes the foundation and defines how the brain will work for the rest of your child's life. Nerve structure grows and gets covered with *myelin*, creating a system that will decide how your child thinks and feels even throughout their adulthood. The connections and the occurring changes can affect the following:

- Attention
- Memory
- Learning
- Sensory systems
- Processing speed
- Ability to plan and multitask
- Ability to control mood and impulses

The surroundings and how you nurture and take care of your child are crucial for these connections and changes.

Breastfeeding your child can make a huge difference as breast milk is the first perfect food for your child while establishing a closer mother-child connection.

As your child grows, there are certain nutrients that are very important for the healthy brain development of your child.

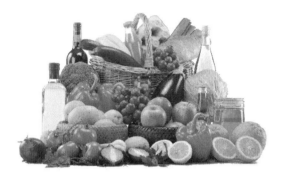

BRAIN NUTRITION

It has long been proven that there is a direct link between diet and brain health. What we eat has significant effects on our brain.

Now that we are aware that food plays an important role not only in making our children strong and healthy but also in developing in them smarter brains, we have to know the right kind of food to feed them.

So what are the foods that can sharpen memories and make learning easier for them?

To optimize brain power, Debra Burke of the Franklin Institute came up with a dietary guide that focuses on the basic food groups.

. . .

Protein

This nutrient is found in meat, poultry, seafood, eggs, soy products, beans and peas, dairy, and nuts and seeds.

Fats

We always hear that nuts will make you intelligent. There's truth to this as our body needs **essential fatty acid** (EFA) which can be found in seeds and raw or roasted nuts. Avocados, extra virgin olive oil, and fresh coconut are also great sources of EFA.

Another excellent source of EFA is meat, but as much as possible get meat from free-range animals or animals that are raised naturally. Free-range animals are allowed to graze in open fields so their diet of grasses is rich in EFA.

Carbohydrates

Our brain needs glucose to fuel all areas into functioning properly. Without enough fuel, we can feel weak and lack concentration, which is why it is better to eat small meals frequently instead of eating three heavy meals in a day. Foods that are rich in carbs are:

- Potatoes
- Corn
- Winter squash
- Beets
- Whole grains
- Cereals
- Crackers

However, consuming foods that are rich in carbohydrates can increase our sugar levels which can be corrected when combined with protein sources including:

- Soy burger with corn
- Salmon with potato
- Egg with potatoes
- Salmon with hash potatoes

MICRONUTRIENTS

Fruits and vegetables have high levels of micronutrients needed by our body and brain. They have antioxidant properties to protect us from free radicals, which are the usual cause of most diseases and disorders.

For our body to have enough of the required daily allocation, nutritionists recommend five servings of fruits and veggies. However, for cancer patients, this amount is usually increased to 9-10 servings.

The role of food in brain health is significant especially when the brain exhibits signs of mental disorder. A common example is depression. Although there are accepted medical treatments for depression, the importance of food and nutrition as incorporated in treatments are widely recognized. This is important since people who are depressed generally have lost their appetite. Therefore, when a person is showing depression symptoms, fast foods and artificial foods are the first to go, along with alcohol, white flour products, simple carbohydrates, caffeine, and artificial sweeteners.

Getting rid of these foods will help improve the chemical balance of the brain. It's best that you keep burger and French fries out of your meals as they are responsible for blocking arteries and small blood vessels, interfering with the blood flow.

VITAMINS

B Vitamins

The four most important vitamins are B1, B6, B12, and folic acid.

People over 60-69 have a 25% deficiency in **Vitamin B12** and a 40% deficiency for those over 80 years of age. It is due to the decline in hydrochloric acid as a person ages. Hydrochloric acid is responsible for breaking down B12 in the digestive system. Deficiency in B12 leads to cognitive decline including poor memory, decrease in reasoning abilities, and mood functions.

Vitamin B6 is responsible for converting stored blood sugar into glucose and is the brain's only fuel. It also protects blood vessels and there are studies saying that it prevents heart attack. As one reaches middle age, he will need 20 percent of Vitamin B6 compared to younger people to maintain efficient cognitive functions. While it promotes blood circulation, it is essential to memory improvement. Vitamin B sources are fish, potatoes, and other starchy vegetables and fruits that aren't citrus, liver, and other organ meats.

Thiamine or B1 is a powerful antioxidant and influences metabolic processes in the brain and central nervous system. However, too much intake of alcohol may deplete B1.

Folic acid is another important substance under B Vitamins. When it comes to depression, folic acid plays a vital role as lower levels of folic acid can result in more serious depression.

Vitamin C

Vitamin C has antioxidant properties that can improve longevity. It is associated with building neurotransmitters such as dopamine, acetylcholine, and norepinephrine while enhancing cognitive abilities.

Vitamin D

Vitamin D is considered the sunshine vitamin and the best way is to get it from sunshine before it gets too hot. You can also get Vitamin D from the flesh of fatty fishes like salmon. Other sources include fish liver oil and fortified products like fortified milk.

Vitamin E

Vitamin E is recognized as the brain aging phenomenon as it is supposed to delay the aging process. It also has antioxidant properties like Vitamin C and can help improve the brain's cognitive abilities when taken with selenium.

Minerals

Magnesium

People who are depressed also show signs of deficiency in magnesium. Magnesium supplements with calcium help a depressed individual not to over-react when stressed and panicked.

Potassium

Most often, we don't need a potassium supplement as it is the most abundant mineral found in the body. Foods like bananas, potatoes, and orange juice are rich in potassium. However, before taking a potassium supplement, it is important to consult with your physician, especially when you are on medication.

Zinc

This mineral plays a key role in the brain's metabolic processes as it protects the brain by destroying free radical molecules in the brain while sparing neurons from damages. Oysters have the most zinc content but can also be found in meat, nuts, fish, and dairy products,

Other brain foods are amino acids, glutamine, tryptophan, and arginine.

Glutamine enhances clarity of thinking and provides mental alertness.

Tryptophan is considered the "feel good" neurotransmitter.

Arginine – this is naturally converted into **spermine** – a chemical that helps in processing memories.

SLEEP

A good night's sleep always makes us feel good and it is the same with children. Not only will sleep give your child's body time to rest and recharge, but it is also crucial to the brain's ability to learn and remember.

Since your body is on rest while you sleep, your brain finds the time to process all information gathered from the day and store them in your memories. Hence, if your child is deprived of quality sleep, they are at risk of developing serious health problems and the inability to learn. Their ability to retain new information may likewise be impaired.

FRESH AIR

Getting fresh does make us feel better but most of us are not aware of how fresh air affects the brain.

Oxygen is absolutely essential in many ways - in maintaining a healthy brain, for growth function, and healing. The fact is, our brain uses about three times as much oxygen as muscles do for healthy neuron functions and are sensitive to decreases in oxygen levels. So, when a person breathes fresh air, it actually improves brain function.

De-Stress

It is common for children to feel disorganized and forgetful when under a lot of stress. However, if children are subjected to stress for a long period, stress may change their brain in ways that could affect their memory. Stress can not only affect memory but can also affect mood, develop anxiety, and promotes inflammation which can harm the heart health of children.

Meditation

Meditation is the process of practicing presence and calming the mind. It is one of the healthiest activities that parents can provide to their children. With meditation, children can process information more clearly. Meditation also affects different parts of the brain, especially in the parietal lobe. This because activity involving the parietal lobe slows down during meditation.

The benefits of meditation, both physically and mentally, are now widely recognized even in children. According to Catherine Wilde of Kids Yoga and Meditation, children too can feel overwhelmed with information they are receiving daily so that learning meditation can be beneficial for them.

BRAIN-BOOSTING FOODS – 10 BRAIN FOODS TO SUPERCHARGE YOUR CHILD'S BRAIN PERFORMANCE

Certain foods are sure to help your child get smarter and do better in class. These are brain foods that help boost the brain and improve your child's brain functions as well as their concentration and memory. Here are 10 foods that will supercharge your child's performance at school.

Salmon

Salmon is rich in omega-3 fatty acids - DHA and EPA. These two substances are essential for brain growth and functions. Research proves that people who have enough fatty acids in their diets develop better mental skills.

So, instead of preparing tuna sandwiches for your children, you can switch to a salmon salad for sandwiches or salmon patties. While tuna is likewise a source of omega-3 fatty acids, it's not as rich as salmon.

Eggs

Choline is an important nutrient that your kids need for memory development. This substance is found in the yolk of an egg. An egg is an excellent source of protein. You may give your child a breakfast of scrambled egg, boiled egg, or an egg sandwich for breakfast before going to school.

Peanut Butter

Peanut butter can be a delicious spread for sandwiches or dips for fruits and veggies like bananas and celery. Children enjoy eating peanut butter, which is a good thing because it is rich in Vitamin E - an antioxidant that protects nerve membranes. Peanut butter also contains thiamine and glucose. Thiamine is best for the brain while glucose is the energy for the brain and body.

WHOLE GRAINS

When the brain needs the energy to fuel it, it's glucose that does the work. Sources of glucose are whole grains like cereals and bread. Whole grains are rich in Vitamin B which is good for the nervous system.

Simply add cereals to your child's breakfast and it is sure to boost your child's brain.

OATS AND OATMEAL

These foods are the best energy provider for your child's brain. Packed with fibers, oats help children stop food cravings and prevent them from eating junk foods for snacks. Oats are also good sources of Vitamin E, B complex, and zinc which optimizes brain performance.

Oatmeal with fruits like bananas, apples, almonds, and blueberries are loved by children.

BERRIES

Known to improve memory, berries are good for your children. They have antioxidant properties that fight free radicals and are packed with Vitamin C. Seeds from berries are rich in omega-3 fatty acids essential for brain functions.

Give your child berries - cherries, blackberries, and blueberries. Berries are healthy snacks and can be a healthy, delicious ingredient of a cool, refreshing smoothie.

Beans

Although commonly known as good for the heart, beans are likewise good for the child's brain and are rich with protein, fiber, complex carbs, vitamins, and minerals. They can keep your child's energy level on heights. Pinto and kidney beans contain more omega-3 fats compared to other beans. As we already knew, Omega-3s fatty acids are essential for brain growth and function.

Vegetables

Colorful vegetables are excellent sources of antioxidants to keep your child's brain healthy and alert. So, always remember to include sweet potatoes, tomatoes, carrots, pumpkins, kale, spinach, and cucumber into your children's meals. If your children don't like to eat veggies, it's easy to sneak them into soups or spaghetti. You may also use the magic of spiralizer in your preparation of vegetable dishes.

Milk And Yogurt

B Vitamins, which are found in enzymes and dairy products, are badly needed by the brain for the growth of brain tissues and neurotransmitters. Children and teens need a higher amount of Vitamin D than adults, and dairy is an excellent source of Vitamin D.

Yogurt and low-fat milk are also good sources of protein and carbohydrates for the brain.

. . .

Lean Beef Or Meat Alternative

Lean beef, or any meat alternative, is rich in iron. Iron helps your children maintain their focus and concentration while in school.

Beef contains zinc, which is good for memory. For children who love to eat vegetables, black beans and soy burgers can be good options for beans contain non-heme iron. However, for non-heme iron to be absorbed, it needs Vitamin C. So, when preparing veggie burgers or beans for your children, partner them with orange juice or include peppers which are good sources of Vitamin C.

CHAPTER 8

SKILLS ESSENTIAL IN CHILD'S LEARNING

THERE ARE different skills essential to our everyday living that we need to continue developing. The ability to think, visualize, and focus on something is basic to us humans that developing them is crucial to what you will be and where you will be in the future. These skills somehow determine your ability to decide and solve the problems you encounter.

Even children need these skills in their learning processes. To help your children develop these skills, you have to understand each of these skills to be able to guide your child in their learning development.

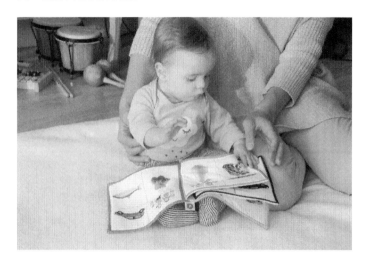

CRITICAL THINKING

Critical thinking is a clear and reasonable reflective thinking focused on deciding what to do or believe in. It involves asking the 4 *Ws* (**what, why, when, and where**) and **how** questions to arrive at a certain decision. It involves many challenging assumptions instead of merely accepting someone else's idea.

If you want your child to excel in their learning, they must learn how to think. Although teaching them to read and write in addition to memorization and fluency in languages may help, they are not enough. We want our children to have flexible minds that can readily absorb new information and decide what's best; we need to develop their critical thinking skills.

But how can we encourage our children to think critically when they are still too young?

Encouraging your children to be inquisitive – e.g. is to ask the question – in a field where they are experts; you will help develop this much-needed skill of critical thinking.

Even when you're too busy with something, do not discourage your children from asking questions. If you don't have the time or the focus to answer them, encourage them to explore for the answer but never make them feel they are neglected. Furthermore, encourage your children to report what they had learned from school and from there, ask them questions that go beyond the "what" like "why" and "how" to develop their inquisitiveness in school.

By asking to children how they came to know the answer, they will learn to justify it which requires them to reflect on their answer to support it. Also, make your child aware that how they see things could be different than how other people see it. For example, when your child talks to you about animal poaching, ask them why people are poaching and how it can affect nature and people in general.

Finally, you can ask them how to solve the problem. You will be surprised at how children will answer your question. Children learn faster than adults because their prefrontal cortex, where working memory is stored, is developed more quickly at this point. In adults, they begin to develop functional fixedness where adults see everything exactly as they are. Let's say, an adult can see a broomstick as it is, while from a child's viewpoint they can see it like a javelin stick. This is due to the creativity produced by their prefrontal cortex, giving them the ability to be inventive and flexible.

It is likewise fascinating to know that children can be very creative and constantly discover new things.

Therefore, by encouraging your children to be inquisitive, it would be a great way to help them develop their skills and talents while still very young.

Critical thinking is not just for children. This is applicable even for adults. We can also improve our critical thinking skills by asking a few questions each day.

ANALYTICAL THINKING

To solve problems, we often break them down into smaller chunks so it will be easier for us to deal with them piece by piece. We call this analytical thinking. It allows children to solve complex issues by filtering through relevant information and identifying patterns and trends. It is a significant skill that everyone needs to achieve success in school, at work, and throughout life.

How To Develop Analytical Thinking Skills

Let Them Solve Math Problems

Solving problems is a common and easy way to improve analytical skills. Math depends on logic, and mathematical problems are structured in ways that children are given a certain amount of information. The problem must be solved using only the provided information. You may correlate everyday life with math problems and allow your children to solve them.

Provide Them with Learning Opportunities

Children learn through exploration and discovery. Providing them with more tools and resources will help them get a better understanding of the world and this understanding will help them solve problems. Resources could be in the form of books, newspapers, videos, science magazines, or community classes. There is a vast range of information that one can easily reach via the internet, but make sure that you are properly guiding your children when using these unlimited resources of information.

Encourage Your Child to Play Brain Games

Playing brain games is a fun way to develop your child's analytical skills and brainpower. By encouraging your child to think in a logical structure, you are providing them an important foundation necessary in facing challenging problems. It is an excellent way to develop their logical reasoning while enjoying the fun.

VISUALIZATION

Visualization is a technique to help your child create images, diagrams, or animation to relay a message. Using visualization through images, visuals, and graphics has been an effective way to communicate concrete and abstract ideas.

In learning, visualization is a cognitive tool that accesses imagination to realize all aspects of action, object, or result.

For children who are struggling to read, visualization can help them create a mental picture that is critical for processing and absorbing information. This mental imaging is a component of the visual process.

Often we find children who have vision problems and cannot visualize or create images in their heads. However, once corrected, there can be a significant improvement in reading.

Here is the best method to help your child learn the skill

of visualization. Show them a picture and allow them to examine it for about 5 minutes. After the allotted time, ask your child to draw what they have seen.

FOCUS/CONCENTRATION

Some children are struggling to pay attention in class and having a hard time completing homework and class activity due to lack of focus and concentration. Issues like these can have a big impact on a child's performance at school.

There can be many reasons why a child finds it hard to focus – it could be from organization problems or comprehension. What is important is that it is possible to help your child improve their focus and concentration.

Tell Them to Do One Thing at a Time

For children with issues on focus and concentration, multitasking is a problem. Jumping between activities causes them to lose momentum. To avoid this, train your child to do one thing at a time instead of working on many things at once. This will teach them to focus only on what is before them rather than thinking of many other things which only leads them to accomplish nothing.

Break Things Into Smaller Pieces

Some tasks become unmanageable for children so teach them to break big tasks into smaller ones to improve their focus as things become manageable for them.

.   .   .

Create a To-Do List

Study sessions, homework, assignments, and projects can be overwhelming to a child. Sometimes it's not because of lack of focus but because they do not know what to focus on. So before he starts to tackle any assignment or study session, create a to-do list for your child to serve as his guide. After your child is able to achieve each task, allow a short break to ready his brain for the next one.

Clear the Study Area

A disorganized study area can be a major source of distraction for your children so make sure that it's cleared of any discomfort or disturbance. It must include only items that will be needed while working on their tasks.

Organize Notes and Notebooks

Organized notes are equally important in an organized study area. Teach your child how to organize their notes to find things quickly. They may use color tabs or coding for every subject.

Also, make sure that your child's notes are neat and complete by checking it every day right after class.

Unorganized notes can take more time, which could have been spent on tasks, and it can also represent an added distraction to the child.

Learning How to Deal with Distractions

Distractions can be everywhere and you can't completely safeguard your child from all distractions.

However, you can train your child to avoid them. Mindfulness techniques, which are a form of meditation, is one of the best ways to teach your child to gain focus.

CHAPTER 9

5 WAYS YOU CAN IMPROVE YOUR CHILD'S MEMORY

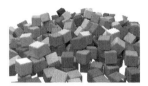

When teaching your child something, it is natural for you to assume that your child can understand everything you taught them. However, this is not always the case. When you teach, there are three possible results:

- Your child absorbs and remembers everything and has a meaningful learning experience
- Your child absorbs and remembers just some portion of the lessons
- Your child learned nothing at all from what you have taught

Ideally, you want your child to learn everything, but if he is struggling in reading or spelling, it's time that you consider revising your concept of teaching by learning these 5 ways to improve your child's memory.

THE FUNNEL CONCEPT

When your concept of teaching it proved to be ineffective, instead of thinking about an eventually unobstructed channel between you and your child, think of a funnel. The funnel has a bigger opening but a smaller end. When you are teaching your child, the information passes through a channel that forms like a funnel.

When you pour too much information, only a small portion passes through until the end or it can get clogged. The same thing works with your child's brain. When you provide your child with too much information, usually the tendency is that the information retained by the memory is only a portion of what you have provided. We call this "information overload" and when instead short-term memory isn't overloaded, the result is increased learning.

MAKE CONNECTIONS

Your child's brain continues to reorganize, adapt, and restructure. New information is added while your child learns. So to help your child, you can teach him to organize information so he can retrieve it later more easily.

Knowledge is organized in networks known as "schemas". As your child adds more information to his knowledge base, this schema is getting more and more complex. Added knowledge may include:

- Sounds of letters
- Which letters are vowels and which are consonants
- How to spell a word
- How to blend sounds to read a word and then

later, a sentence, and so on. Every bit of information added is connected to something that is already there. Therefore, if the new information does not relate to anything that has been stored, then it can't be stored in long-term memory and the information is simply dropped.

If you want to help your child build a schema, there are simple and effective ways to do it.

Building Connections To Things They Previously Knew

For example in spelling, if you are confused about when to use ie against ei, just remember the name Alice. When the letter that comes before is the letter "l", use the vowel "ie" but when it's letter "c", what follows is "ei".

Example: receipt, receive, relieve, believe

Using Analogy

An analogy is comparing two different things. An example would be when teaching syllable types. You may use "door" for an "open syllable". An open syllable has no consonant to close it like in he, the, me, tree, free, etc.

Providing Content With Unifying Themes

This is grouping items using themes. An example is using colors as codes like yellow for vowels and red for consonants.

Another example is grouping animals or grouping

plants so your child can identify if a dog is an animal or a plant.

By helping your child build organized schema, you are helping him establish long-term memory.

As they add new information bit by bit, each piece of this information is connecting to something that has already been there and this is what makes your teaching more effective. Even as information is growing, because they are well-organized, your child can easily recall them later when needed.

THE SMI METHOD

The SMI method (Simultaneous Multisensory Instruction) is a special subset of multi sensory teaching.

If your child can't remember what you're teaching, it is not because something is wrong with his memory but it might be the way you're teaching.

It's normal to believe that learning starts in the brain, but the truth is it starts with your child's senses. Senses are pathways to the brain, and when teaching you are engaging different pathways: sight, touch, and sound.

However, in traditional teaching, spelling is taught using the visual pathway and leaving the other major pathways behind when we could have had to make use of sound (auditory) and movements (kinesthetic) pathways to the brain. Using all these pathways can be extremely beneficial to your child's learning.

Remember that your child's senses are in charge of gathering information and sending it to his brain, and it is their brain deciding whether to process them or not. If the brain approved, it will store this information in their short-term memory for further processing. Therefore, the more receptors that are involved, the better the chances that the brain will retain this information.

MAKE LEARNING STICK

Another way to make reading and spelling stick in your child's memory is by making learning imprinted in his memory.

Let me explain better...

In this method of teaching, the review is a critical component. Most often a review is not often stressed in most curriculums but to make sure that your child has the mastery of his lessons, you have to be consistent and include a review. You can't assume that what you taught him will automatically stick to his memory. To implement this method there are review strategies you must consider adopting.

Make sure that your child understands the main point of what you're teaching. If you are teaching your child about prefixes, then make clear that your goal is to learn about prefixes.

In teaching about prefixes, you are teaching your child to add a prefix before the root word. Your child will be learning what prefix and root words are.

You must demonstrate clearly how to attach the prefix word to the root word. Remember that your child must clearly understand the lesson before you can proceed with reviewing the lesson.

The review is incorporated with the lesson.

As you proceed to a new lesson, have a quick review of the lesson previously taught to ensure that he remembers doing it.

Review more often when a new concept is first taught.

When teaching a new concept or idea and you fail to review it from time to time, there's a great chance that your child will easily forget it. So make sure that you review it daily at first until it is imprinted in your child's memory.

As your child masters it, the review activity will be less and less as you introduce a new concept to learn. Reviewing lessons this way pushes information into long-term memory where it is kept for later recall.

Certain concepts are reviewed using the same words until your child had completely mastered it.

IMPROVE WORKING MEMORY

Did you ever notice your child easily forgets things when you send them on an errand? This inability to remember even a short list of tasks demonstrates the shortcomings of your child's working memory. For a child with more memory challenges, this can have a significant impact on their learning process. Before we begin to discuss ways to improve or enhance your child's working memory, let's take a moment to define it first.

WHAT IS WORKING MEMORY

Working memory is the capability of your brain to hold information for a short period while you are processing this information. Working memory is crucial for learning to read and spell.

Here are some of the things where working memory can help:

- It helps you remember the words as you read

through a sentence or a paragraph for better comprehension

- It helps you sound out unfamiliar words
- It helps you remember where you are in the text you're reading, even if you left for a while and return soon
- It allows you to compose content through a series of sentences – making you think of what to write next while you're writing

Working memory can be an indicator of how a child can learn.

Signs To Spot That Your Child Has Poor Working Memory

Children with poor working memory face difficulties with tasks that require them to hold information in their minds, such as dictated sentences, while struggling with the spelling of some words. It may appear that the child is not paying attention, but the truth is, he simply forgot the initial part of the sentence dictated that he has to write down.

Moreover, a child with poor working memory may be facing any of the following issues:

- Difficulty paying attention to lessons
- Seems uncooperative during learning activities
- Finds it hard to comprehend what they are reading
- Often forgets what they want to say
- Often misplaces things
- Seems forgetful
- Struggles to complete multi-step activities

- Can't follow a string of instructions

IMPROVE YOUR CHILD WORKING MEMORY

To help your child improve their working memory, try doing the following ideas.

Avoid too much information. Once there is information overload presented in a lesson, children with poor working memory tend to be distracted or stop taking in information.

Minimize Distractions. Try reducing distractions when your child is working. Children can easily get distracted when there is a TV or radio in the background or when other children are talking or doing interesting activities.

Provide comfort. Children easily get stressed when learning is not fun and enjoyable. Stress in children can manifest in forms of headaches, hunger, feeling too hot or cold, eye strain when there are vision issues, or when facing a bright window. Stress can harm your child's working memory.

Read aloud every day. Reading aloud allows your child to recall what you have just read and to anticipate what's following. While listening to your loud voice he is interpreting each word and understands the story you are reading. Have this activity for 20 minutes every day.

Simplify instructions. Do some simple activities with your child that requires him to follow instructions like doing crafts or cooking simple recipes. Allow him to read the simple instructions and let him do the steps. Just make sure that the instructions are within your child's level of comprehension. Doing this exercise will stretch the child's working memory.

Play games that encourage the building of memory skills. Games like matching and concentration are great options to play with your child.

Be encouraging to your child. To minimize stress, be patient and be encouraging. Note that children do not want to disappoint you so they worry about their performance and this will only create a negative impact on their working memory.

CHAPTER 10

DEVELOPING YOUR CHILD'S MINDSET

LINGUISTIC INTELLIGENCE

Linguistic Intelligence, in its simplest meaning, deals with an individual's ability to communicate. To help your child develop this skill, try to incorporate some of these activities into your child's daily life:

- Singing
- Role-Play
- Alphabet Games
- Storytelling
- Playing word games

When your child is four years old and can write, teach them to express their feelings through writing. Encourage them to draw and illustrate their thoughts and then ask them to explain what they have drawn.

Other activities you can provide to a four-year-old child and older are:

- **Keeping a journal**. Allow your child to keep a journal. It is very helpful in organizing, processing emotions and experience, and making sense of what is happening around them.

- **Indulge them in discussions and debates.** This means to involve your child in positive conversations on different topics to create in them awareness and interest.

- **Ask them to maintain a scrapbook**. Teach your older children to create a scrapbook. It is a creative way to develop writing skills through highlighting events, interviews, creative writing, pictures and captions, illustrations, and many more.

- **Teach your child new words each day**. Introduce new words every day to your child. This will not only develop his vocabulary but also develops their potential to be a word warrior as they grow older. Finding new words to include in the scrapbook and the conversation can be a fun way of building your child's vocabulary.

SPATIAL INTELLIGENCE

Spatial skills are essential for success in various areas and industry ranging from Physics to Engineering and Visual Arts. Although your child's intelligence has something to do with genetics, still it is clear that learning experiences can greatly influence it.

Moreover, it can predict their achievement in Science,

Mathematics, Engineering, and Technology. Spatial skills are likewise critical for visual artists, mechanics, surgeons, and architects.

Unluckily, traditional schooling provides little opportunities to foster the development of spatial abilities in our children. However, studies indicate that people can improve their spatial skills with training (Dewar, n.d.).

FLUID INTELLIGENCE

Teaching your child to think critically? You might wonder if your child is capable of critical thinking and will work it out by themselves. After all, we are all able to think logically even without formal lessons in logic.

Furthermore, studies have shown that children can become better learners once they are given the opportunity to explain how they solve problems.

HELPING YOUR CHILD DEVELOP A GROWTH MINDSET

"I can't understand Mathematics, so how can I answer this?" If you hear your child saying something like this, it is not about motivation or resiliency, but it could be about a growth mindset.

A growth mindset believes that intelligence and abilities continuously develop throughout a person's life and can be strengthened through concentrated practice and effort.

In simple terms, it describes how your child faces challenges. A growth mindset is opposed to a fixed mindset which believes that their abilities can't be changed regardless of their effort.

Having a growth mindset can have its benefits as it helps your child reframe their approach to challenges.

This concept of Growth Mindset was developed by Carol Dweck, a psychology professor at Stanford University who believed that there are two kinds of mindset: the growth mindset and fixed mindset. According to her, children who face challenges believe they can improve but those who pulled back believe they couldn't (Rippel, 2020).

For example, if your child believes that he can't answer his exercises because he finds math difficult, then he has a fixed mindset. But if he chooses to learn math and studies hard, that is growth mindset. Having a growth mindset means more than just accepting feedback and being open-minded but it is also learning from feedback and experience. A person with a growth mindset believes that failure isn't the end of everything for you because you always have the chance to improve and succeed. With that, they can come up with strategies for improvement.

Children need to know that failures can be turned into strengths, so encourage your children to speak up when something is wrong or when they need help. They also need to know that you believe they can find a way to fix their mistakes. You may tell your child, "It is alright, you can do it next time if you study harder!"

Take note that a growth mindset is an ongoing process. It is a continuous process of receiving feedback from others and applying it for improvement while learning from mistakes. This way, children are learning to find ways to approach tasks they find difficult at first. It's a valuable way for children to learn that talents can be developed and skills can be learned.

CHAPTER 11

BRAIN GAMES & COGNITIVE STIMULATION EXERCISES

Learning is supposed to be fun and enjoyable for children and not limited to books and boring activities in school. The best ways to motivate your child to learn are simple and fun activities that can help stimulate and accelerate their verbal and motor skills. Here are some games and exercises that you should expose your child to at the earliest stage. These are recommended for children between 2-5 years of age.

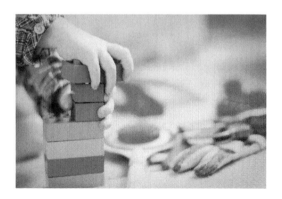

Building Blocks

Every child should start with this most basic game. For this game, you will need a set of blocks with each side of different colors and images. With building blocks, you can introduce a variety of themes or groups like shapes, animals, plants, letters, and numbers.

This is one of the most basic games that has evolved over the years but has never faded out. All you need are a set of blocks, preferably in different colors and shapes, leaving the rest up to your child's imagination.

Puzzles

A puzzle is one game you can't risk missing and have to start as soon as possible as an older child may ignore it for more exuberant games. This game helps improve hand-eye coordination to logical reasoning and on top of it is the confidence boost that comes from completing the puzzle. While it develops better self-esteem in children, it likewise deters procrastination in them.

Memory Cards

Memory cards are best for exercising your child's memory recall with fun. They are available on physical cards and via digital devices.

There is a wide range of memory games to choose from online, so choose a comfortable and suitable level for your child.

Encourage them to move on to more tiles as they get better. Opt for ones with interesting features like those with different shapes, characters, and icons.

. . .

Word Hunt

This will teach your child to form words using alphabets either in cards, blocks, or magnets to form different words. Then with the use of flashcards ask your child to match them.

For example, the word in the card is a DOG. Ask your child to form the same word using blocks or cards.

Role-Playing

Role-playing is great in boosting the imagination and creativity of children. They can portray the role of a doctor, nurse, teacher, witch or anything they can think of. The activity can also help set the right moral tone for your child and will benefit them as they adjust to their environment and society.

Beading and Sewing

These two activities are good for the development of your child's fine motor skills and also a good exercise for their brain. In beading, let them use beads of different colors, shapes, and sizes. Instruct them to follow a certain pattern like three yellow round beads, and then four green stars, six white flowers, and so on. Let them get engrossed with the activity and their final reward could be a bracelet they made out of those beads.

For children that are 7-8 years of age, teach them to sew on a plastic canvas that doesn't require sharp needles and following a pattern. They can sew pouches and clutches out of this engaging activity while improving their cognitive abilities. Through this activity they are required to follow precise instructions that are very easy and yet the result will provide them with a good and enjoyable learning activity.

Finding Things

It is a fun way of introducing your toddlers to their environment – either at home, in the park, or at school.

Show your child an image of an object, let's say of a BALL, and ask them to find it. You may also teach your child the right pronunciation and object recognition through this activity side by side with cognitive development.

Mazes

This is an effective way of teaching children to follow directions like:

- Three steps forward
- Go right or left
- Go ahead
- Turn back
- To the right

This game is a big hit for kids that addresses a variety of skills, aside from being a perfect brain-boosting activity. You may also use a variety of maze books available in bookstores and on the internet.

The maze game can provide your child with the following advantages:

- Visual-motor skill development – your child will start the game by scanning throughout the page to figure their way out of the maze. The ability to scan is needed in reading and writing.

- Fine motor skill development – this activity requires your child to draw a line for the direction they will take without touching the side. Your child must learn to control the pencil with his fingers.
- Problem-solving ability – the child needs to find their way into the maze and out of it which can be confusing given the many options.
Developing the ability to solve a problem is crucial in everyday life.

Matching Objects

This game is recommended for toddlers between 2-4 years old.

Images in the first column must match with images on the next column. For example:

- Bee – Honey
- Rain – Raincoat
- Pitcher – Glass
- Cup – Saucer
- Baby – Diaper

This is a great opportunity for you to teach your child about pairing while strengthening concepts they previously learned. Vary themes like using rhyming and opposite words. You may also match words with actions or senses with things like Taste – Food, Hear – Music, See – TV, etc.

Texture Play

Playing using senses can stimulate your child and his brain. Exploring things around them using their senses can keep their brain active and helps build more neural pathways. Teaching children how to sense textures is vital as they can't just learn them by reading books. It involves actual experiencing and trying it out with various objects around and can be a delightful activity for children who are just starting to explore their environment and learn from it. Allow children to play with different things and feel every object with their hands; like sand, walls, slime, clay, etc.

CONCLUSION

Your Children's education is of vital importance and that's why you invest in their schooling. As parents, you can't just depend on educators for your child's learning, growth and development. Understanding all their needs, including learning needs, is one of the basic responsibilities of parenting.

While a child's major means of learning is through exploring, they also learn on their own through their senses – sight, sound, smell, taste and touch. Our responsibility as parents is to enhance this learning experience by providing a positive environment, primarily at home, where they spend most of their time growing and developing their brain.

After reading this book, I expect you to have a greater understanding of the importance and roles parents play in helping form a child's brain, both for a better working memory than memory recall.

Now that you are aware of the most effective tools to

improve your child's memory and can make the difference in their learning process, you must put this knowledge into practice.

All you have to do is stimulating your child's memory in a playful way by creating a positive and child-friendly learning environment. Also, you must endeavor to keep strengthening their successes and minimizing their mistakes.

In doing so, they will remember more and more every day.

Offering our child the best tools to improve their memory can be really a great fulfillment in our parenting journey, but above all, it will guarantee them a bright future.

Our children's success lies in our hands and it is our fundamental task as parents to see that they succeed in every aspect of their lives. The keys and knowledge of what we can do for them is imprinted on the pages of this book. I hope that you found it helpful because I wrote it with the only purpose of helping you improve your child's future.

Now, you just need to put these tips into practice. I wish you all the best!

"Your memory is the glue that binds your life together; everything you are today is because of your amazing memory. You are a data collecting being, and your memory is where your life is lived."

KEVIN HORSLEY

ONE LAST THING...

REVIEW PAGE

If you enjoyed this book or found it useful, I'd be very grateful if you'd post a short review. All you need to do is just click the link below or scan the code and share your thoughts. It is quick and painless and will only take a second.

Thanks again for your support!
Lisa Marshall
Click HERE to leave a Review

OTHER BOOKS

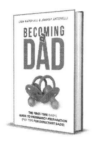

Becoming a Dad
The First-Time Dad's Guide to Pregnancy
Preparation (101 Tips For Expectant Dads)

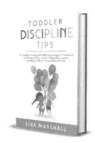

Toddler Discipline Tips
The Complete Parenting Guide With Proven
Strategies to Understand And Managing
Toddlers' Behavior, Dealing With Tantrums,
And Reach An Effective Communication
With Kids

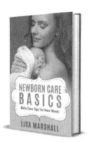

Newborn Care Basics
Baby Care Tips For New Moms

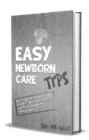

Easy Newborn Care Tips
Proven Parenting Tips For Your Newborn's
Development, Sleep Solutions And Complete
Feeding Guide

FREE GIFT

Thank you for purchasing this book! Click on the link to download your FREE gift!

https://bit.ly/childlearningstylez

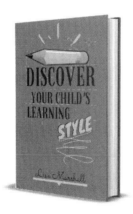

By understanding your child's preferred learning style you can:

- Improve your child's accomplishments and feelings of achievement
- Teach your child coping skills for situations that are not geared to their learning style
- Help your child at home thanks to the best tools

And much more!

DO YOU ENJOY AUDIOBOOKS?

1. If you prefer to learn by listening, be sure to check out my audiobooks! You can listen for FREE if you're a first time Audible user as part of their free 30-day trial.
2. Click the link and enjoy your next audiobook!

https://bit.ly/enjoyaudiobooks

REFERENCES

Bernard, S. (2010, December 1). Neuroplasticity: Learning Physically Changes the Brain. Retrieved from https://www.edutopia.org/neuroscience-brain-based-learning-neuroplasticity

Cunningham, A., & Stanovich, K. (1998). What Reading Does for the Mind. American Educator. (22). Retrieved from https://www.researchgate.net/publication/237109087_what_reading_does_for_the_mind

Dana Foundation. (2010, August 16). Brain Scientists Identify Links between Arts, Learning. Retrieved from https://sharpbrains.com/blog/2009/05/24/brain-scientists-identify-links-between-arts-learning/

Dewar, G., PhD. (n.d.). Spatial intelligence: What is it, and how can we enhance it? Retrieved April 6, 2020, from https://www.parentingscience.com/spatial-intelligence.html

Dweck, C. (2007). Mindset: The New Psychology of Success (1st ed., Vol. 1). Retrieved from https://www.amazon.com/gp/product/

Hanna, J., PhD. (2017, May 13). What Educators and

Parents Should Know About Neuroplasticity, Learning and Dance. Retrieved from https://sharpbrains.com/blog/2016/01/22/what-educators-and-parents-should-know-about-neuroplasticity-learning-and-dance/

Learning languages is a workout for brains, both young and old | Penn State University. (2014, November 12). Retrieved from https://news.psu.edu/story/334349/2014/11/12/research/learning-languages-workout-brains-both-young-and-old

Leopold, W. (2007, November 13). Early Academic Skills, Not Behavior, Best Predict School Success: Northwestern University News. Retrieved from https://www.northwestern.edu/newscenter/stories/2007/11/duncan.html

Michelon, P. (2018, April 9). Brain Plasticity: How learning changes your brain. Retrieved from https://sharpbrains.com/blog/2008/02/26/brain-plasticity-how-learning-changes-your-brain/

Rippel, M. (2020, March 24). Improving Your Child's Working Memory + Downloadable E-book. Retrieved from https://blog.allaboutlearningpress.com/improving-working-memory/

Santos, E. (2020, April 6). Synaptic Pruning. Retrieved from https://link.springer.com/referenceworkentry/10.1007%2F978-0-387-79061-9_2856

St. Louis, M. (2020, February 6). How to Spot Visual, Auditory, and Kinesthetic-Learning Executives. Retrieved from https://www.inc.com/molly-reynolds/how-to-spot-visual-auditory-and-kinesthetic-learni.html

Steele, C. J. (2013, January 16). Early Musical Training and White-Matter Plasticity in the Corpus Callosum: Evidence for a Sensitive Period. Retrieved from https://www.jneurosci.org/content/33/3/1282

Weiner, S. (2017, December 8). Why Do Domesticated Animals Have Tiny Brains? Retrieved from https://www.popularmechanics.com/science/animals/a14392897/domesticated-brains/

Who's (Socially) Smarter: The Dog or the Wolf? (2017, December 10). Retrieved from https://www.sciencemag.org/news/2013/05/whos-socially-smarter-dog-or-wolf

Printed in Great Britain
by Amazon

50267919R00076